Sensei Self Development

Mental Health Chronicles Series

Exploring Your Spiritual Beliefs

Sensei Paul David

Copyright Page

Sensei Self Development - Exploring Your Spiritual Beliefs, by Sensei Paul David

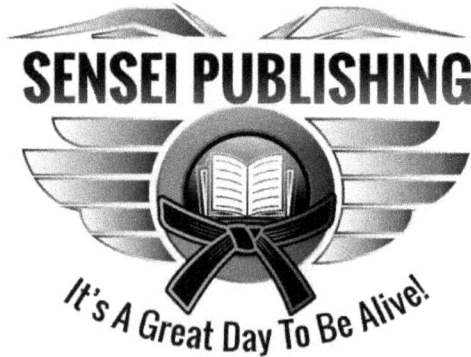

SENSEI PUBLISHING

It's A Great Day To Be Alive!

www.senseipublishing.com

@senseipublishing
#senseipublishing

Get/Share Your FREE SSD Mental Health Chronicles at
www.senseiselfdevelopment.care

or

CLICK HERE

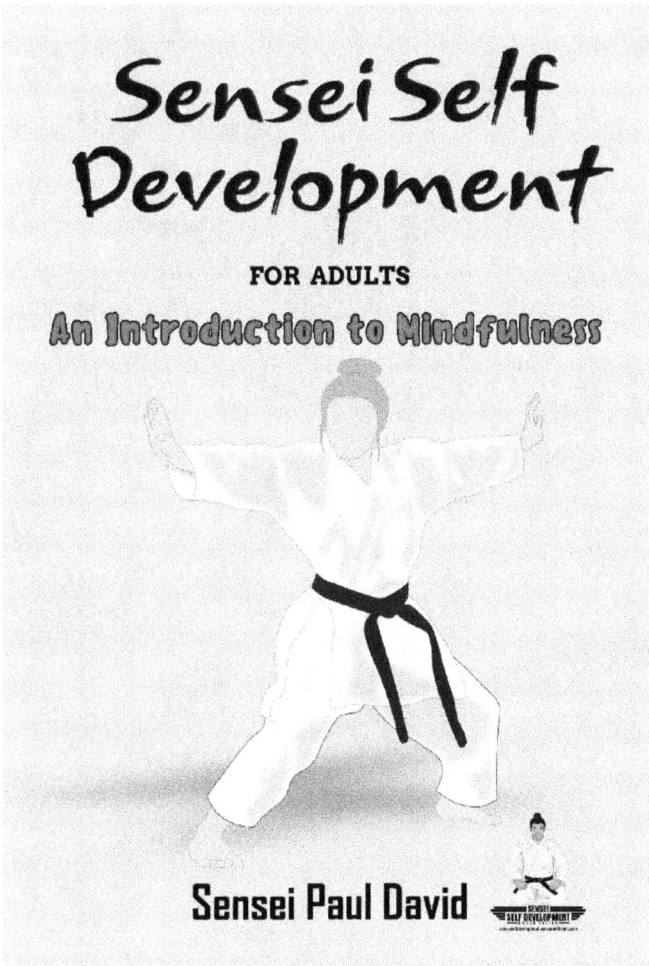

Check Out The SSD Chronicles
Series CLICK HERE

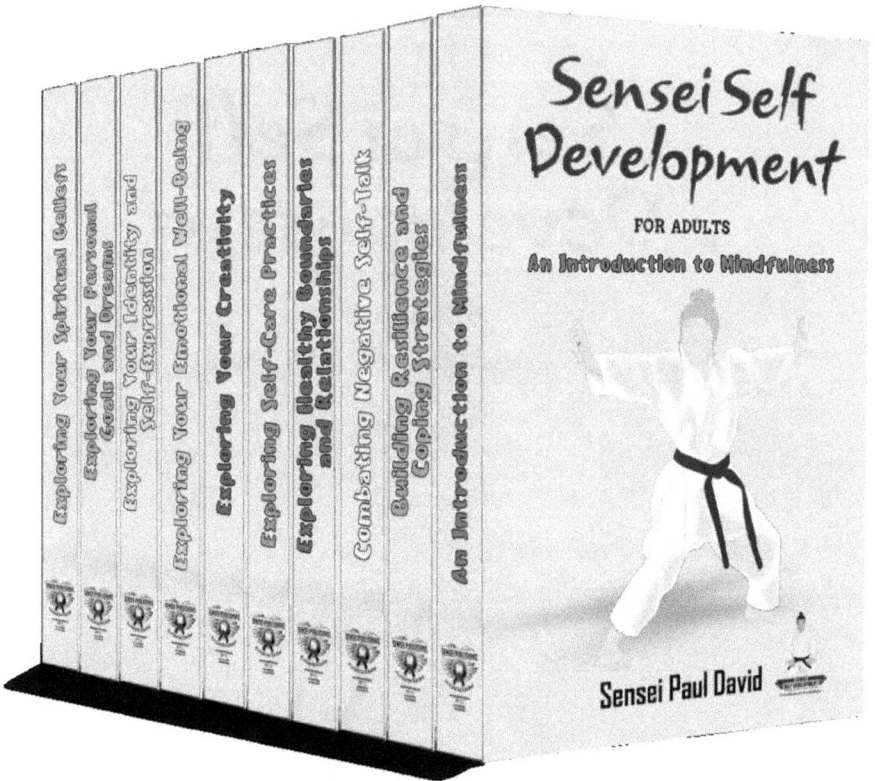

Exploring Your Spiritual Beliefs

Exploring Your Personal Goals and Dreams

Exploring Your Identity and Self-Expression

Exploring Your Emotional Well-Being

Exploring Your Creativity

Exploring Self-Care Practices

Exploring Healthy Boundaries and Relationships

Combatting Negative Self-Talk

Building Resilience and Coping Strategies

An Introduction to Mindfulness

Sensei Self Development

FOR ADULTS

An Introduction to Mindfulness

Sensei Paul David

Dedication

To those who courageously take action towards self-improvement - you are helping to evolve the world for generations to come.

- It's a great day to be alive!

If Found Please Contact:

_____

Reward If Found:

_____

MY
COMMITMENT

I, _____
commit to writing This Sensei Self Development Journal for at least 10 days in a row, starting: _____

Writing this journal is valuable to me because:

_____

_____

_____

_____

_____

_____

If I finish a minimum of 10 consecutive days of writing in this journal, I will reward myself by:

_____

_____

_____

_____

_____

_____

If I don't finish 10 days of writing this journal, I will promise to:

_____

_____

_____

_____

_____

_____

I will do the following things to ensure that I write in my Sensei Self Development Journal every day:

_____

_____

_____

_____

_____

_____

Get/Share Your FREE All-Ages Mental Health eBook Now at

www.senseiselfdevelopment.com

Or CLICK HERE

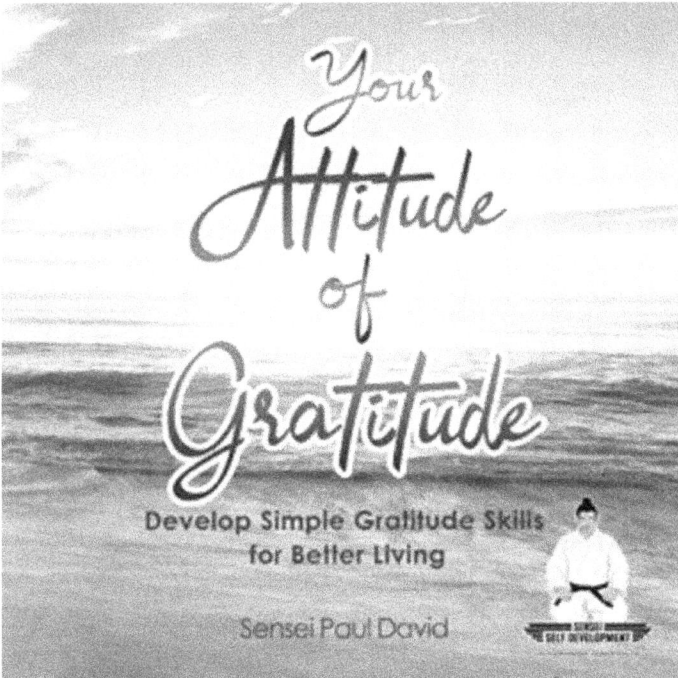

senseiselfdevelopment.com

Check Out Another Book In The
SSD BOOK SERIES:

senseipublishing.com/SSD_SERIES

CLICK HERE

SENSEI
SELF DEVELOPMENT
BOOKS SERIES

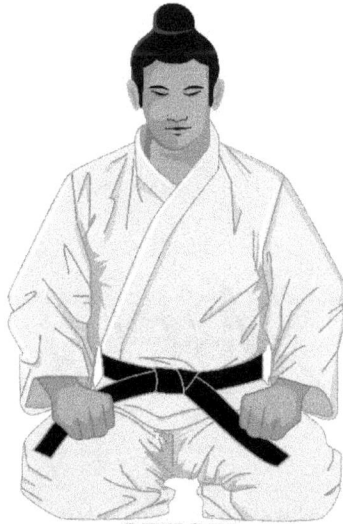

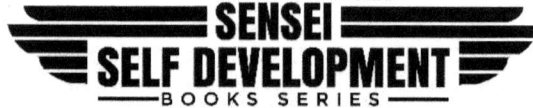

senseiselfdevelopment.senseipublishing.com

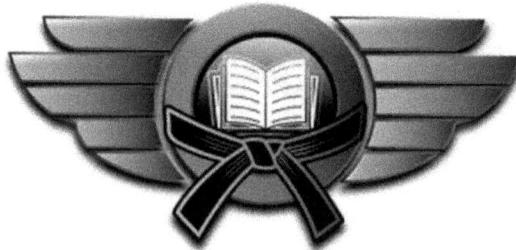

Join Our Publishing Journey!

If you would like to receive FUTURE FREE BOOKS and get to know us better, please click www.senseipublishing.com and join our newsletter by entering your email address in the pop-up box.

Follow Our Blog: senseipauldavid.ca

Follow/Like/Subscribe: Facebook, Instagram, YouTube: @senseipublishing

Scan the QR Code with your phone or tablet

to follow us on social media: Like / Subscribe / Follow

A Message From The Author:
Sensei Paul David

Dear Reader,

Welcome to the world of mental health journaling — a sacred space for self-reflection, growth, and healing. Within these pages, you hold the power to uplift your spirit, invigorate your mind, and nourish your goals.

In a world that often moves at blink-and-you'll-miss-it speed, it's crucial to make time for self-care and self-discovery.

Anxiety, stress, and emotional turbulence may have clouded your mind, making it difficult to find clarity and peace within. But fear not! Together, we will navigate the labyrinth of emotions, and experiences, helping to simplify the path to mental well-being.

This journal is not merely a bunch of blank pages awaiting your words. It is your compassionate companion, offering solace and understanding during your unique journey. Here, you are free to unburden yourself, celebrate small and large victories, and confront the challenges that may still linger.

Within the sheltered realm of these pages, there is no judgment, no expectation, and no pressure. Your unique experience and perspective hold immeasurable worth, and your voice deserves to be heard. Whether you choose to fill the lines with eloquence or simply scribble fragments of your thoughts, please remember each entry is a valuable contribution to your growth.

In this sacred space, you are challenged to take off the mask we so often wear in the outside world. It is here that you can be raw, vulnerable, and authentic – allowing your true self to be seen and embraced without reservation. By giving yourself permission to explore the depths of your emotions and confront the shadows that may lurk within, you will discover profound insights and find the healing you seek over time.

As you embark on this journaling journey, I encourage you to embrace the process itself rather than fixate solely on the outcome. Remember, it is not about reaching a certain destination or ticking off boxes on a list of accomplishments. Rather, it is about cultivating self-awareness, fostering self-compassion, and nurturing a sense of curiosity about the intricate workings of your intelligently beautiful mind.

In the quiet moments of reflection, let your pen become a bridge between your inner world and the possibilities that lie ahead. Create a sanctuary for your thoughts, fears, triumphs, and dreams. As you pour your heart onto these pages, allow your words to be a living testament to courage, resilience, and an unwavering commitment to your own well-being.

I am honored to be a part of your journey, and I believe in your ability to navigate the twists and turns with grace and resilience. Remember, you are not alone in this – countless others have walked similar paths, faced similar challenges, and emerged stronger and wiser on the other side. You have the power to reclaim all of your untapped joy, cultivate a positive mindset that serves you, and foster a deep sense of self-love and peaceful confident. – And it will take a worth effort and time.

So, open the first page of this journal with hope, curiosity, and an open heart and open mind. Embrace the transformative power of self-reflection, and allow it to guide you towards a life of greater fulfilment and peace. Each journaling session is an opportunity to not only connect with yourself but also to rekindle the light within that sometimes flickers but never extinguishes.

Remember, the pages you are about to fill are not just a record of your journey but also a testament to your strength, resilience, and indomitable spirit. Cherish this space, invest in yourself, and let your words be an ode to the magnificent journey of becoming whole.

With great respect for your decision to evolve,

Paul

MY CONVICTION

Please circle your answers below

I am DECIDING to be patient with myself and this PROCESS each time I journal toward my improved state of mental well-being

YES   NO

"The present moment is filled with joy and happiness. If you are attentive, you will see it."

Thich Nhat Hanh

Introduction

Spiritual Beliefs

Recently, traditional religious practices have significantly declined in America, particularly among younger generations. Surveys reveal that Millennials and Gen Z adults are more likely to have no religious affiliation compared to older generations, leading to what's called "the rise of the 'nones.'" While some view this as a sign of societal decay, others see it as progress.

However, it's less often noted that Americans are still more inclined than those in other developed countries to engage in religious or spiritual activities, such as daily prayer, without adhering to a specific religion. A 2017 Pew Research Center survey found that only about 18 percent of Americans consider themselves neither spiritual (believing in something transcendent or sacred) nor religious (affiliated with specific religious groups). A significant 48 percent identified as both religious and spiritual, while another 27 percent claimed to be spiritual but not affiliated with any religion. (Just 6 percent considered themselves religious but not spiritual.)

The fact that spirituality still thrives in the U.S. surprises many in social sciences. They've long thought that as society becomes more focused on data, technology, and science, people would move away from spiritual beliefs.

But looking closer at recent studies, it's not so shocking that spirituality remains strong. Whether it's through traditional religion or other forms of spiritual practice, these experiences offer something special. They give us insights into life and benefits that you just can't get from anything else. Putting aside the arguments about whether religious beliefs or spiritual experiences are right or real, it's clear that exploring these spiritual aspects can help people understand life better, feel happier, and love more deeply.

People often turn to religious and spiritual practices to find meaning in a world that can be confusing. They might realize that understanding life's deeper meaning isn't something they can find in their regular routines or in worldly pursuits like entertainment or material consumption. Many are also searching for experiences that feel 'bigger' than everyday life – moments of awe, a connection with others or the divine, or a sense of transcending the usual boundaries of space and time.

These experiences aren't just figments of our imagination; they have a strong basis in our brain's workings. Research shows that our brains respond in specific ways to religious and spiritual experiences. Psychologist Lisa Miller, who wrote "The Awakened Brain," has extensively studied the brain's role in spiritual experiences. For instance, she found that recalling a spiritual experience, as opposed to a stressful one, reduces activity in the medial thalamus and caudate. These are areas linked with sensory and emotional processing. This suggests that spiritual experiences might help people break free from overthinking and constant rumination. Other researchers, looking at patients with brain lesions, have connected self-reported spirituality to activity in the periaqueductal gray. This area of the brainstem is involved in moderating fear and pain and is associated with feelings of love.

The research is undeniable. Spirituality makes us experience reality differently and that experience, or that way of being, is unlike anything that we can get from something other than spirituality. Worldly pleasures such as winning a championship or having sex may feel good, but they are fundamentally different from spiritual experiences – which tend to be deeper and longer lasting.

Benefits of Spiritual Beliefs

Focusing specifically on the impact of spiritual beliefs (as opposed to practices or community involvement), scientific research has highlighted several areas where these beliefs can positively influence an individual's well-being:

1. Resilience in Face of Stress: Belief in a higher power or a greater purpose can offer a broader perspective on life's challenges, aiding individuals in coping with stress and adversity.

2. Sense of Purpose and Meaning: Spiritual beliefs can provide a strong sense of meaning and purpose in life. This can lead to greater life satisfaction and can be particularly helpful in times of crisis or loss.

3. Positive Outlook and Optimism: Some studies suggest that those with spiritual beliefs may have a more optimistic outlook on life and a greater expectation of positive outcomes.

4. Coping with Illness and End-of-Life Peace: For patients facing serious illnesses or end-of-

life issues, spiritual beliefs can provide comfort, reduce fear of death, and help in making sense of difficult situations.

5. Moral and Ethical Guidance: Spiritual beliefs often come with a set of moral or ethical guidelines that can help individuals make decisions and navigate complex social and personal situations.

6. Connection and Interconnectedness: Beliefs in interconnectedness or a universal spirit can foster a sense of unity with others and the world, promoting feelings of compassion and empathy.

It's important to note that the impact of spiritual beliefs can be very personal and subjective, and the scientific study of these effects often involves complex, nuanced methodologies to account for a wide range of variables.

Interconnectedness of all Things

The concept of interconnectedness has long been a topic of fascination for thinkers across various fields - philosophy, science, and spirituality. It proposes a fundamental connection between all elements of the universe, from minuscule particles to immense galaxies, suggesting that our choices and actions have wider implications than we might realize.

A prominent figure who deeply contemplated this idea was Marcus Aurelius, the Roman emperor and philosopher. In Meditations, he muses, "All things are implicated with one another, and the bond is holy; there is hardly anything unconnected with any other thing." This statement emphasizes that everything in the universe is part of a larger, interconnected system, and our actions and choices are not isolated events, but integral parts of this vast network.

Interconnectedness isn't just a philosophical notion; science, particularly quantum physics, supports it too. In the quantum realm, phenomena like electrons and photons are intertwined in ways that defy conventional understanding, famously termed as "spooky action at a distance." This concept, known as quantum entanglement, illustrates that actions on one particle can have immediate effects on another, even across vast distances, measured in light years.

The idea of interconnectedness is found across various spiritual traditions in the world. One notable example is the Native American belief in the "web of life," which underscores the need to live harmoniously with nature.

Moreover, the idea of interconnectedness has practical applications in our personal lives. Understanding that everything is interconnected can lead us to live with more compassion, empathy, and mindfulness. It reminds us that our actions and choices impact not only our immediate surroundings but also the broader world, including future generations. By recognizing our role in this interconnected web, we can make decisions that benefit not just ourselves but the larger community and environment.

Ways to Apply the Concept of Interconnectedness in Our Day-to-Day Lives:

1. Acting with a Sense of Responsibility Towards Future Generations: Making decisions that consider the well-being and prospects of those who will come after us.
2. Living in Harmony with Nature: Acknowledging our impact on the environment and striving to reduce it, thereby living more sustainably.
3. Practicing Empathy and Understanding Towards Others: Recognizing how our actions impact others and cultivating a

sense of empathy and understanding in our interactions.

4. Cultivating Gratitude for Interconnected Resources: Appreciating the interconnected nature of both material and immaterial resources we use in our daily lives.

5. Considering Long-Term Consequences of Our Actions: Making decisions with an awareness of their long-term effects, beyond immediate outcomes.

6. Developing an Attitude of Interconnectedness in Relationships and Community: Fostering a sense of unity and collective well-being in our personal relationships and community engagements.

The idea of interconnectedness is deeply rooted in various philosophical, scientific, and spiritual teachings. It teaches us that everything in the universe is interlinked, and our choices and actions can significantly impact the broader world. Understanding our role in the web of life encourages us to live with greater compassion, empathy, and understanding. This awareness not only benefits us individually but also contributes positively to those around us and the world at large. As Marcus Aurelius insightfully noted, "All things are implicated with one another, and the bond is holy." Embracing this interconnectedness is key to leading more meaningful and fulfilling lives.

Self is an Illusion

Many of us have a tendency to let negative emotions linger longer than necessary. When we become angry, for instance, we often sustain this anger by dwelling on the reasons for it. This process involves actively recalling the insult or event that sparked the anger, but we rarely notice how we're perpetuating these feelings. If we stop fueling the anger, it naturally dissipates in a short time.

Meditation can teach us not to remain in a state of anger for an extended period. The difference between being angry for a few moments versus hours or days is significant. Even without meditation, we've all experienced interruptions in our negative emotions, like suddenly having to switch to a pleasant demeanor for an important phone call. These interruptions are natural experiments in mood shifts, showing how quickly we can change our mental state by shifting our focus.

However, you don't need to wait for a distraction to change your mood. By paying close attention to your negative emotions without judgment, and observing their nature and effects on your body, you can understand how they vanish on their own.

Thinking is crucial for our human capabilities, but our constant identification with thoughts leads to suffering and the illusion of a separate self living inside our heads. Try to stop thinking for a minute and you'll notice how challenging it is. This difficulty points to the extraordinary fact that, without substantial meditation training, maintaining awareness even for a short while is nearly impossible.

Being continuously lost in thought, as most of us are, is seen in Eastern contemplative traditions as the source of suffering. Thoughts aren't the problem; it's our identification with them that causes issues. Meditation helps break this identification, allowing us to see thoughts as fleeting and not integral to our sense of self.

Through meditation, you can understand that the feeling of "I" is just a product of thought, a temporary state in consciousness. The goal is to recognize the moments between thoughts, to see the selfless nature of consciousness. Just like the optic blind spot, the selflessness of consciousness is always present, yet often unnoticed. With practice, however, one can learn to see consciousness as it is: free of the self and a mere witness to our thoughts and emotions.

Belief in Higher Power

Belief in a higher power generally refers to the idea that there's a supreme force or entity beyond our physical universe. This entity is often seen as supernatural, existing outside the natural laws of the universe. In many cultures, this higher power is credited with creating and sustaining the universe, and is often viewed as a moral authority, setting guidelines for human behavior. Beliefs about this power can vary; it might be a personal being, like in monotheistic religions such as Christianity, Islam, and Judaism, or an impersonal force, as seen in some Eastern philosophies. This belief is deeply tied to personal faith and spirituality, providing comfort, purpose, and a sense of connection to something greater. Across cultures and religions, there's a rich diversity in how this higher power is understood and related to. Some emphasize its transcendence, being entirely beyond the physical world, while others focus on its immanence, or presence within the world and individuals. Regardless of the details, belief in a higher power provides numerous benefits to the believer.

Believing in a higher power can offer numerous benefits. It often brings a sense of comfort and solace, especially during challenging times, giving people a feeling that they're not alone in their struggles. It's been linked to better mental health, as studies show that people with strong spiritual beliefs often have lower rates of depression and anxiety. This belief can provide a coping mechanism during stress, offering a sense of hope and resilience.

Belief in a higher power can provide a strong sense of purpose and meaning in life, answering big questions about existence and our role in the universe. For many, it fosters a sense of community and belonging, as shared beliefs bring people together in religious or spiritual groups. It can also offer moral guidance, helping individuals determine right from wrong based on teachings attributed to a higher power. This belief can encourage personal growth and resilience, as people often turn to their faith in times of crisis or change. It can also promote compassion and empathy, as many faiths emphasize the importance of caring for others. For some, the belief in a higher power leads to experiences of awe and wonder, appreciating the mystery and beauty of the universe. It can also encourage a sense of humility and gratitude, acknowledging the limits of human understanding and being thankful for life's blessings. Additionally, for many, this belief provides a framework for understanding and accepting life's mysteries and uncertainties, offering a sense of peace in the face of the unknown.

Belief in the Idea of Spiritual Enlightenment

Enlightenment is a profound alteration in how one perceives and understands reality. It's not just about temporary changes in state or emotion but a fundamental shift in the structure of perception itself. This transformation allows for a deeper, more holistic grasp of reality, transcending typical boundaries of individual consciousness.

Contrary to common beliefs, enlightenment doesn't necessarily lead to perpetual happiness or bliss. It's not an escape from the human condition but a deeper engagement with it. Enlightenment encompasses the full range of human emotions and experiences, integrating them into a broader understanding of existence. This state doesn't erase personal flaws or challenges; enlightened individuals may still face their own struggles and emotional complexities.

A key aspect of enlightenment is the experience of a unified state of consciousness. This means perceiving oneself and the external world as interconnected, breaking down the usual barriers between self and others. It's a recognition of a deeper unity in all aspects of existence, where the distinction between subject and object is transcended.

In essence, enlightenment is about a deep, enduring change in one's understanding of reality. It's a state that integrates all facets of human experience, offering a unique perspective on life and existence. While it might not provide all the answers, it represents a significant shift in consciousness that can have a profound impact on an individual's life.

All spiritual traditions also offer insights as to how one can achieve spiritual enlightenment. Here are some:

1. Meditation and Mindfulness: This is fundamental for calming the mind, increasing awareness, and fostering a deeper connection with oneself and the universe. Regular meditation helps in understanding and controlling thoughts and emotions, leading to greater inner peace and enlightenment.
2. Self-Reflection and Personal Growth: Introspection is crucial in understanding oneself, one's purpose, and one's place in the universe. This involves regularly examining one's thoughts, beliefs, and actions, and striving for personal growth and self-improvement.

3. Compassion and Service: Many spiritual traditions teach that true enlightenment involves transcending self-centeredness and serving others. Acts of kindness, empathy, and service to others can cultivate a sense of connectedness and universal love.

4. Study and Learning: Engaging with spiritual texts, teachings, and philosophies can offer guidance and insight on the path to enlightenment. This includes learning from the wisdom of various spiritual traditions and applying their teachings in daily life.

These four pillars can serve as a solid foundation for anyone seeking spiritual enlightenment.

Suffering Provides Meaning to Life

While our instinctual drive leans towards seeking pleasure and avoiding pain, cultural attitudes play a significant role in shaping how we approach suffering. In the Western world, there's a tendency to view suffering as an obstacle to happiness, leading to efforts to fight, suppress, or quickly fix it. However, in many Eastern traditions, suffering is recognized for its crucial role in personal growth and the path to enlightenment.

Tibetan monk Khenchen Konchog Gyaltshen Rinpoche identifies four benefits of suffering: the cultivation of wisdom, resilience, compassion, and a profound respect for reality.

Wisdom, as noted, often emerges from suffering. When life is smooth, we seldom pause to reflect deeply. It's through adversity that we're jolted into a state of introspection, leading us to develop what King Solomon called a "wise heart."

Echoing this sentiment, Friedrich Nietzsche famously stated, "What does not kill us makes us stronger." Suffering can build our resilience, much like muscles that grow stronger through exertion. Helen Keller, who experienced both joy and suffering, observed, "Character cannot be developed in ease and quiet. Only through experience of trial and suffering can the soul be strengthened, vision cleared, ambition inspired, and success achieved."

Compassion is another byproduct of suffering. As the dictionary defines it, compassion is a deep awareness of the suffering of another coupled with the wish to relieve it. This deep awareness is often born from our own experiences of pain. Pastor Fritz Williams notes, "Suffering and joy teach us, if we allow them, how to make the leap of empathy, which transports us into the soul and heart of another person."

Suffering also instills a deep respect for reality. While joy connects us to the realm of possibilities, pain reminds us of our limitations. It's a humbling experience that contrasts the highs of ecstasy, where we often look upwards, dreaming of the infinite, with the lows of agony, where we look downwards, grounded in the finite.

This perspective on suffering doesn't imply that we should seek it out. Just as we don't actively seek illness to strengthen our physical immune system, we don't need to seek suffering to fortify our psychological resilience. The imperfections and transience of the world naturally present us with enough challenges to strengthen our emotional fortitude.

The Buddha's First Noble Truth acknowledges the inevitability of suffering in human existence. When we learn to accept and even embrace life's difficulties, our suffering becomes a tool for personal growth. This acceptance transforms our adversities into instruments for developing deeper understanding and resilience.

Present Moment is All There Is

Everything you've ever experienced, thought, or felt has happened in the present moment, the Now. Can you think of a time when this wasn't the case? Will it ever be? The answer is clear: it's not possible for anything to happen outside the Now.

What we call the past occurred in a Now that has already passed. When we remember the past, we're simply bringing back those past Nows in our current moment. The future, too, is just the Now waiting to happen. When we think about the future, we're projecting our present thoughts forward.

The past and future don't have their own reality. They are like the moon, which doesn't shine by itself but reflects the sun's light. Similarly, the past and future are reflections of the light of the present. They borrow their reality from the Now.

The essence of what I am saying here cannot be fully comprehended by the mind. When you truly understand this concept, there is a shift in consciousness from a mind-dominated state to one of presence and being. It's a transition from being caught up in time to being immersed in the present. Suddenly, the world around you seems alive, vibrant with energy, and emanating a sense of being.

In emergency situations where there's a threat to life, people often experience a natural shift in consciousness from focusing on time to being fully present. The usual personality, with its past and future, momentarily steps back, replaced by a state of intense, conscious presence. This presence is extremely still yet highly alert. The appropriate response to the situation then emerges from this state of consciousness.

This shift is also why some people are drawn to risky activities like mountain climbing or car racing. They may not realize it, but these activities force them into the Now – a state of being intensely alive, beyond time, free from problems, thinking, and the weight of personality. In such activities, losing touch with the present moment, even briefly, can be fatal. However, this dependence on a specific activity to achieve such a state is unnecessary. It's possible to enter this state of intense presence without undertaking extreme challenges like climbing a mountain. You can access it in the here and now.

Throughout history, spiritual masters from various traditions have emphasized the Now as the key to accessing the spiritual realm. Yet, this knowledge often seems like a hidden secret, rarely highlighted in conventional religious teachings. In churches or temples, for instance, you might hear gospel readings like "Take no thought for the morrow; for the morrow shall take thought for the things of itself," or "Nobody who puts his hands to the plow and looks back is fit for the Kingdom of God." You might also encounter teachings about the lilies of the field, which live effortlessly in the present and are bountifully cared for.

However, the true depth and radical nature of these teachings are often overlooked. Few recognize that these messages aren't just philosophical ideas but practical instructions meant to be lived. They're intended to drive a deep, inner transformation, shifting our focus from the burdens of time to the freedom of the present moment.

The core of Zen is about existing entirely in the present moment, the Now. It's about being so fully present that no problem or suffering can persist within you, as they are not part of your true essence. In this state, where time is absent, all your problems simply dissolve. Suffering needs time to exist; it cannot survive in the immediate presence of the Now.

The concept of the Now is crucial in Sufism, Islam's mystical tradition. Sufis express this through the saying, "The Sufi is the son of time present". Rumi, the esteemed poet and Sufi teacher says, "Past and future veil God from our sight; burn up both of them with fire."

Before We Get Started…

Remember, mindfulness journaling is a personal practice, and these questions are meant to guide and inspire you. Feel free to adapt and modify them to suit your needs and preferences. Explore, reflect, and embrace the opportunity to deepen your self-awareness and cultivate a sense of inner peace.

Date ___ / ___ / ___: S   M   T   W   Th   F   S

I feel:
(please circle)

because   because   because   because   because
_____   _____   _____   _____   _____
_____   _____   _____   _____   _____

Today I Am Grateful For

1. _____
2. _____
3. _____

What could help transform today into a remarkable day?

Reflective Writing

What spiritual beliefs do you currently hold?

_____

_____

_____

_____

_____

_____

_____

_____

What does "spirituality" mean to you?

A) Feeling connected to a higher power or the universe
B) Following a specific religious doctrine
C) Having a sense of purpose and meaning in life
D) All of the above

All Are Correct - Choose The Response You Feel Is Most Important To Remember

Date ___ / ___ / ___ : S   M   T   W   Th   F   S

I feel:
(please circle)

because   because   because   because   because
_____   _____   _____   _____   _____
_____   _____   _____   _____   _____

Today I Am Grateful For

1. _____
2. _____
3. _____

What could help transform today into a remarkable day?

Reflective Writing

How has your spiritual beliefs evolved since you were a child?

_____

_____

_____

_____

_____

_____

_____

Which of the following is NOT a form of self-expression?

A) Star of David
B) Cross
C) Crescent moon
D) All of the above

All Are Correct - Choose The Response You Feel Is Most Important To Remember

Date ___ / ___ / ___ : S   M   T   W   Th   F   S

I feel:
(please circle)

because   because   because   because   because
_____ _____ _____ _____ _____
_____ _____ _____ _____ _____

Today I Am Grateful For

1. _____
2. _____
3. _____

What could help transform today into a remarkable day?

Reflective Writing

Do you feel that your spiritual beliefs have a
strong influence on your life?

_____

_____

_____

_____

_____

_____

_____

Which of the following is a common spiritual practice?

A) Meditation

B) Prayer

C) Yoga

D) Mindful breathing

All Are Correct - Choose The Response You Feel Is Most Important To Remember

I feel:
(please circle)

because   because   because   because   because

_____ _____ _____ _____ _____

_____ _____ _____ _____ _____

Today I Am Grateful For

1. _____
2. _____
3. _____

What could help transform today into a remarkable day?

Reflective Writing

What spiritual experiences have you had that have changed your beliefs?

_____

_____

_____

_____

_____

_____

_____

_____

Which of the following is a common approach to spirituality?

A) Rituals and ceremonies
B) Personal reflection and self-exploration
C) Scientific reasoning and evidence
D) Community and social engagement

All Are Correct - Choose The Response You Feel Is Most Important To Remember

Date ___ / ___ / ___: S   M   T   W   Th   F   S

I feel:
(please circle)

because   because   because   because   because
_____   _____ _____   _____   _____
_____   _____ _____   _____   _____

Today I Am Grateful For

1. _____
2. _____
3. _____

What could help transform today into a remarkable day?

Reflective Writing

Do you feel that the spiritual path you are on is
meaningful or fulfilling to you?

_____

_____

_____

_____

_____

_____

_____

_____

Which of the following is a component of spirituality?

A) Connection with a higher power
B) Religious dogma
C) Moral and ethical values
D) Finding inner peace and contentment

All Are Correct - Choose The Response You Feel Is Most Important To Remember

Date ___ / ___ / ___ : S M T W Th F S

I feel:
(please circle)

because   because   because   because   because
_____ _____ _____ _____ _____
_____ _____ _____ _____ _____

Today I Am Grateful For

1. _____
2. _____
3. _____

What could help transform today into a remarkable day?

Reflective Writing

What sources do you rely on for guidance or understanding when exploring your spiritual beliefs?

_____

_____

_____

_____

_____

_____

_____

What is the term for a journey of self-discovery and personal growth often associated with spirituality?

A) Pilgrimage
B) Meditation
C) Enlightenment
D) Soul searching

All Are Correct - Choose The Response You Feel Is Most Important To Remember

Date ___ / ___ / ___ : S M T W Th F S

I feel:
(please circle)

because   because   because   because   because
_____ _____ _____ _____ _____
_____ _____ _____ _____ _____

Today I Am Grateful For

1. _____
2. _____
3. _____

What could help transform today into a remarkable day?

Reflective Writing

How do you feel when you practice your spiritual beliefs?

_____

_____

_____

_____

_____

_____

_____

In which religion is the concept of the Golden Rule ("treat others as you would like to be treated") commonly found?

A) Judaism
B) Islam
C) Christianity
D) All of the above

All Are Correct - Choose The Response You Feel Is Most Important To Remember

Date ___ / ___ / ___ : S   M   T   W   Th   F   S

I feel:
(please circle)

because   because   because   because   because
_____ _____ _____ _____ _____
_____ _____ _____ _____ _____

Today I Am Grateful For

1. _____
2. _____
3. _____

What could help transform today into a remarkable day?

Reflective Writing

How do you differentiate between spiritual beliefs
and religious beliefs?

_____

_____

_____

_____

_____

_____

_____

What is the term for a group of people united by shared beliefs and practices?

A) Congregation
B) Clique
C) Community
D) Collective

A is Correct - Choose The Response You Feel Is Most Important To Remember

I feel:
(please circle)

because   because   because   because   because
_____ _____ _____ _____ _____
_____ _____ _____ _____ _____

Today I Am Grateful For

1. _____
2. _____
3. _____

What could help transform today into a remarkable day?

Reflective Writing

How important is it to you to find alignment
between your spiritual beliefs and your actions?

_____

_____

_____

_____

_____

_____

_____

What is the belief in a higher power or divine being?

A) Agnosticism
B) Atheism
C) Spirituality
D) Theism

D is Correct - Choose The Response You Feel Is Most Important To Remember

Date ___ / ___ / ___ : S   M   T   W   Th   F   S

I feel:
(please circle)

because   because   because   because   because
_____   _____   _____   _____   _____
_____   _____   _____   _____   _____

Today I Am Grateful For

1. _____
2. _____
3. _____

What could help transform today into a remarkable day?

Reflective Writing

What is the role of meditation in your spiritual journey?

_____

_____

_____

_____

_____

_____

_____

_____

In which religion is the concept of Ahimsa (non-harming) central to its teachings?

A) Christianity
B) Buddhism
C) Hinduism
D) Taoism

C is Correct - Choose The Response You Feel Is Most Important To Remember

Date ___ / ___ / ___ : S   M   T   W   Th   F   S

I **feel:**
(please circle)

because   because   because   because   because

_____ _____ _____ _____ _____

_____ _____ _____ _____ _____

Today I Am Grateful For

1. _____

2. _____

3. _____

What could help transform today into a remarkable day?

Reflective Writing

What spiritual practices do you incorporate into
your daily life?

_____

_____

_____

_____

_____

_____

_____

_____

What is the term for a personal set of values and beliefs that guide an individual's actions and decisions?

A) Faith
B) Religion
C) Spirituality
D) Morality

D is Correct - Choose The Response You Feel Is Most Important To Remember

Date ___ / ___ / ___: S   M   T   W   Th   F   S

I feel:
(please circle)

because   because   because   because   because

_____   _____   _____   _____   _____

_____   _____   _____   _____   _____

Today I Am Grateful For

1. _____
2. _____
3. _____

What could help transform today into a remarkable day?

Reflective Writing
Do you have any rituals or traditions that you
follow as part of your spiritual practice?

_____

_____

_____

_____

_____

_____

_____

In which religion is the concept of a moral code based on the Eightfold Path taught?

A) Judaism
B) Islam
C) Buddhism
D) Hinduism

C is Correct - Choose The Response You Feel Is Most Important To Remember

Date ___ / ___ / ___ : S   M   T   W   Th   F   S

I feel:
(please circle)

because   because   because   because   because

_____   _____   _____   _____   _____

_____   _____   _____   _____   _____

Today I Am Grateful For

1. _____

2. _____

3. _____

What could help transform today into a remarkable day?

Reflective Writing
What is the most meaningful spiritual experience you have ever had?

_____

_____

_____

_____

_____

_____

_____

_____

_____

What is the belief that the universe and all its elements have a divine or spiritual essence?

A) Animism
B) Nihilism
C) Agnosticism
D) Dualism

A is Correct - Choose The Response You Feel Is Most Important To Remember

I feel:
(please circle)

because   because   because   because   because
_____ _____ _____ _____ _____
_____ _____ _____ _____ _____

Today I Am Grateful For

1. _____
2. _____
3. _____

What could help transform today into a remarkable day?

Reflective Writing

How do you balance your spiritual practice with the demands of everyday life?

_____

_____

_____

_____

_____

_____

_____

What is the belief that one is responsible for their actions and will face the consequences in this life or the next?

A) A) Karma
B) B) Dharma
C) C) Nirvana
D) D) Enlightenment

A is Correct - Choose The Response You Feel Is Most Important To Remember

Date ___ / ___ / ___ : S   M   T   W   Th   F   S

I feel:
(please circle)

because   because   because   because   because

_____   _____   _____   _____   _____

_____   _____   _____   _____   _____

Today I Am Grateful For

1. _____
2. _____
3. _____

What could help transform today into a remarkable day?

Reflective Writing

What advice would you give to someone just
beginning to explore their spiritual beliefs?

_____

_____

_____

_____

_____

_____

_____

What is the belief that the soul is reborn into a new body after death?

A) Karma
B) Nirvana
C) Reincarnation
D) Salvation

C is Correct - Choose The Response You Feel Is Most Important To Remember

As we reach the final pages of this journey through "Positive Mindset," I want to extend my heartfelt thanks to you. Your commitment to exploring positivity and its transformative power is not only commendable but a testament to your desire for personal growth and a richer, more fulfilling life experience.

Remember, the journey towards a positive mindset is ongoing and ever-evolving. Each day presents new opportunities to apply these principles, to learn, and to grow. I encourage you to revisit these pages whenever you need a reminder of your incredible potential to foster positivity and resilience in the face of life's challenges.

As we part ways, I leave you with a quote that has been a guiding star in my journey: "The greatest discovery of any generation is that a human can alter his life by altering his attitude."

– William James.

Thank you for allowing me to be a part of your journey. May your path be filled with light, hope, and endless possibilities. Farewell, and may you carry the spirit of positivity with you, today and always.

With gratitude and best wishes,

Sensei Paul David

Reflective Writing

_____

_____

_____

_____

_____

_____

_____

_____

_____

_____

_____

_____

_____

_____

_____

_____

_____

_____

_____

_____

The End

As you close the pages of this mindfulness journal, remember that each word you've written is a step on your journey towards self-awareness and inner peace. Embrace the moments of clarity, the revelations, and even the uncertainties you've encountered along the way. Let this journal be a testament to your growth and a reminder that every day offers a new opportunity to be present, to observe, and to appreciate the simple wonders of life. Carry these lessons forward, and may your path be filled with mindful moments and serene reflections. Until we meet again in these pages, be gentle with yourself and stay anchored in the now.

Mindfulness isn't difficult, we just need to remember to do it.

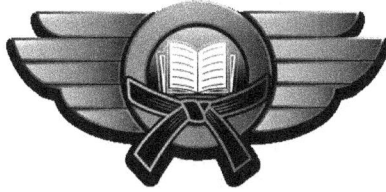

Thank You!

If you found this book helpful, I would be grateful if you would **post an honest review on Amazon** so this book can reach other supportive readers like you!

All you need to do is digitally flip to the back and leave your review. Or visit amazon.com/author/senseipauldavid click the correct book cover and click on the blue link next to the yellow stars that say, "customer reviews."

As always...
It's a great day to be alive!

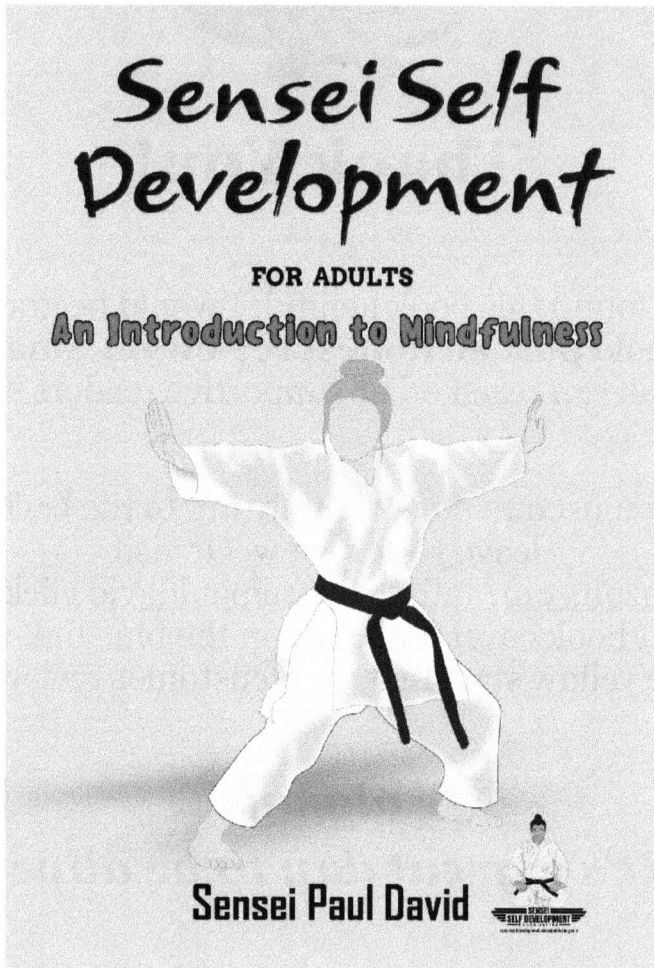

Sensei Self
Development

FOR ADULTS

An Introduction to Mindfulness

Sensei Paul David

Check Out The SSD Chronicles
Series CLICK HERE

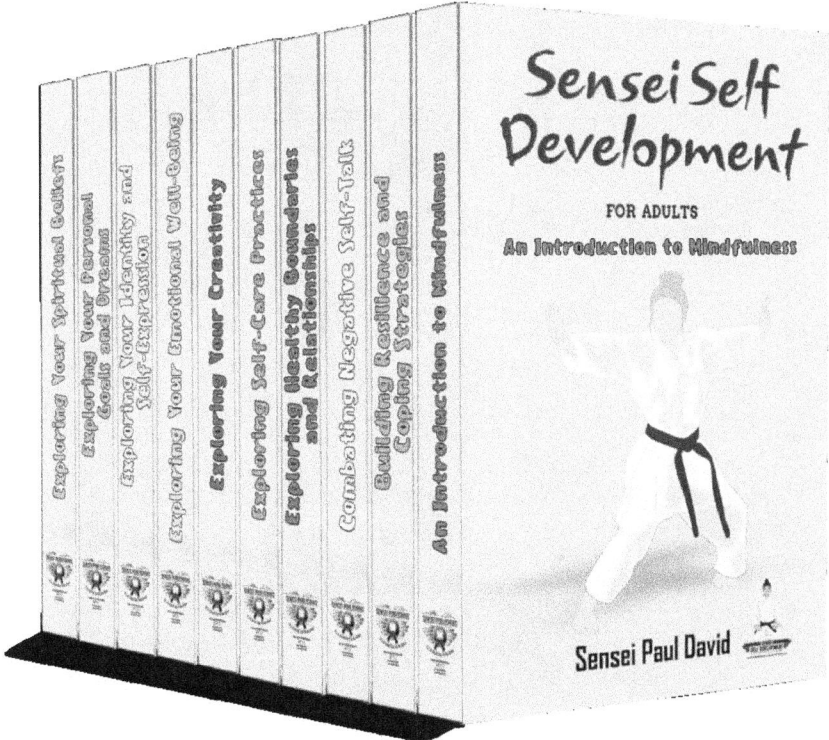

Sensei Self
Development

FOR ADULTS

An Introduction to Mindfulness

Sensei Paul David

Get/Share Your FREE All-Ages Mental Health eBook Now at

www.senseiselfdevelopment.com

Or CLICK HERE

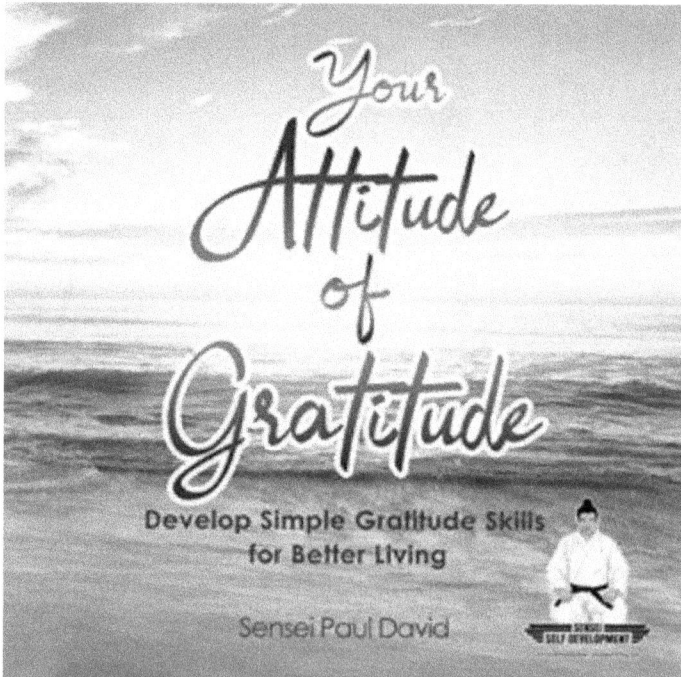

senseiselfdevelopment.com

Click Another Book In The SSD BOOK SERIES:

senseipublishing.com/SSD_SERIES

CLICK HERE

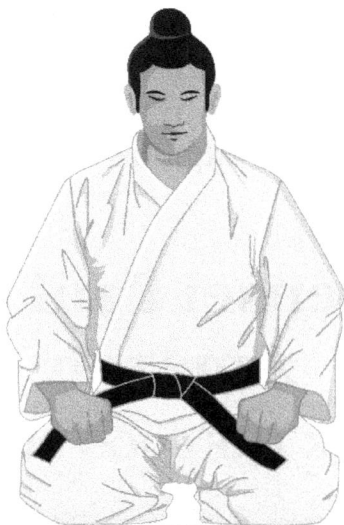

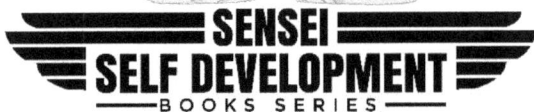

senseiselfdevelopment.senseipublishing.com

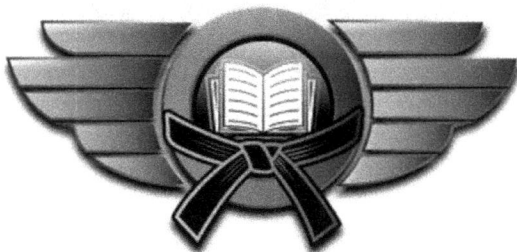

Join Our Publishing Journey!

If you would like to receive FREE BOOKS, please visit **www.senseipublishing.com**. Join our newsletter by entering your email address in the pop-up box

Follow Sensei Paul David on Amazon

CLICK THE LOGO BELOW

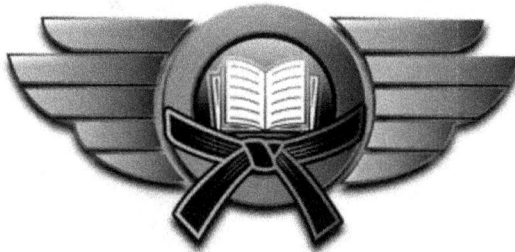

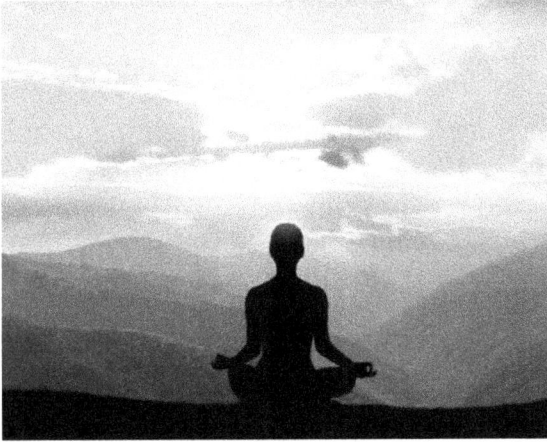

FREE BONUS!!!
Experience Over 25 FREE Engaging Guided Meditations!

Prized Skills & Practices for Adults & Kids. Help Restore Deep-Sleep, Lower Stress, Improve Posture, Navigate Uncertainty & More.

Download the Free Insight Timer App and click the link below:
http://insig.ht/sensei_paul

About Sensei Publishing

Sensei Publishing commits itself to helping people of all ages transform into better versions of themselves by providing high-quality and research-based self-development books with an emphasis on mental health and guided meditations. Sensei Publishing offers well-written e-books, audiobooks, paperbacks and online courses that simplify complicated but practical topics in line with its mission to inspire people towards positive transformation.

It's a great day to be alive!

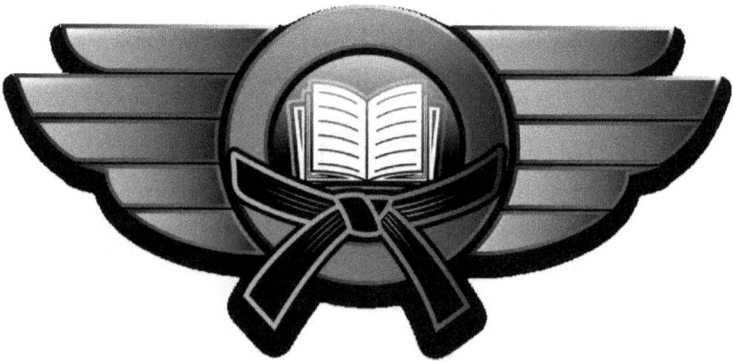

About the Author

I create simple & transformative eBooks & Guided Meditations for Adults & Children proven to help navigate uncertainty, solve niche problems & bring families closer together.

I'm a former finance project manager, private pilot, jiu-jitsu instructor, musician & former University of Toronto Fitness Trainer. I prefer a science-based approach to focus on these & other areas in my life to stay humble & hungry to evolve. I hope you enjoy my work and I'd love to hear your feedback.

- It's a great day to be alive!

Sensei Paul David

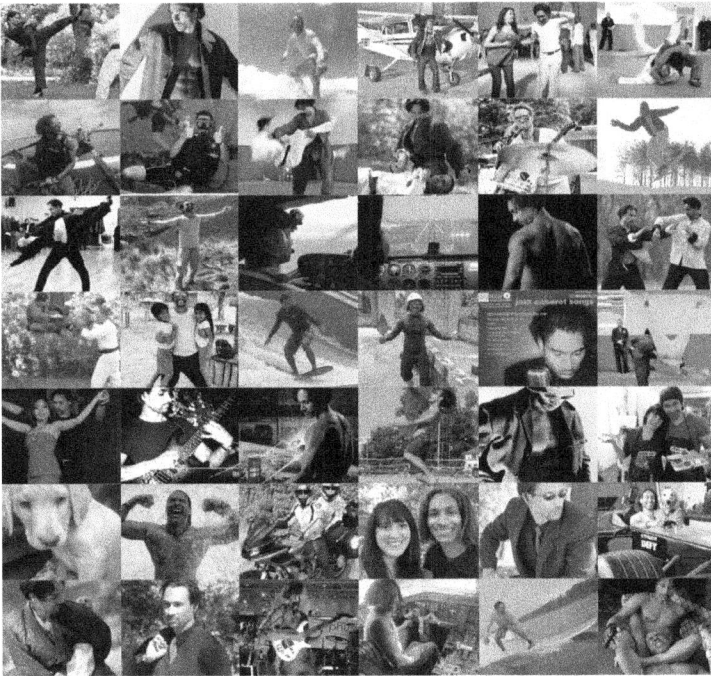

Scan & Follow/Like/Subscribe: Facebook, Instagram, YouTube: @senseipublishing

Scan using your phone/iPad camera for Social Media
Visit us at www.senseipublishing.com and sign up for our
newsletter to learn more about our exciting books and to
experience our FREE Guided Meditations for Kids & Adults.